ALOE VERA

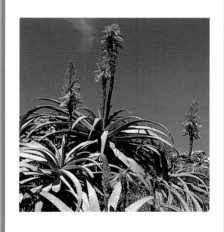

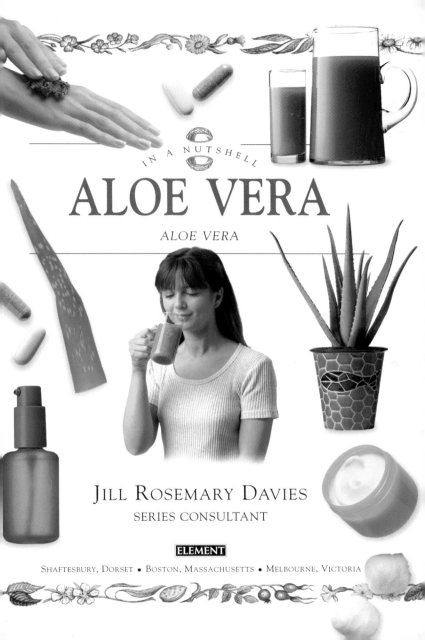

IN A NUTSHELL

ALOE VERA

ALOE VERA

JILL ROSEMARY DAVIES

SERIES CONSULTANT

ELEMENT

SHAFTESBURY, DORSET • BOSTON, MASSACHUSETTS • MELBOURNE, VICTORIA

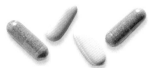

© Element Books Limited, 2000

Series Consultant Jill Rosemary Davies
Text Jill Nice

First published in Great Britain in 2000 by
ELEMENT BOOKS LIMITED
Shaftesbury, Dorset SP7 8BP

Published in the USA in 2000 by
ELEMENT BOOKS INC.
160 North Washington Street,
Boston MA 02114

Published in Australia in 2000 by
ELEMENT BOOKS LIMITED
and distributed by
Penguin Australia Ltd
487 Maroondah Highway,
Ringwood, Victoria 3134

NOTE FROM THE PUBLISHER
Any information given in this book is not
intended to be taken as a replacement for
medical advice. Any person with a
condition requiring medical attention
should consult a qualified practitioner
or therapist.

For growing and harvesting, calendar
information applies only to the northern
hemisphere (US zones 5–9).

Designed and created for Element Books with
The Bridgewater Book Company Ltd.

ELEMENT BOOKS LIMITED
Editorial Director Sue Hook
Project Editor Kate John
Assistant Editor Annie Hamshaw-Thomas
Group Production Director Clare Armstrong
Production Controller Hannah Turner

THE BRIDGEWATER BOOK COMPANY
Art Director Tony Seddon
Designer Jane Lanaway
Editorial Director Fiona Biggs
Project Editor Lorraine Turner
DTP Designer Trudi Valter
Photography Guy Ryecart
Illustrations Michael Courtney
Picture research Liz Moore

Printed and bound in Portugal

Library of Congress Cataloging
in Publication data is available

British Library Cataloguing
in Publication data is available

ISBN 1 86204 709 X

*The publishers wish to thank the following
for the use of pictures:*
AKG London: pp.10t, 19t. Ancient Art
& Architecture: pp.10b, 11b, 12b.
Bridgeman Art Library: pp.8t, 12tl.
ET Archive: p.6tl. Eye Ubiquitous:
p.16b,/James Davis: p.23t. Steven Foster
(www.stevenfoster.com): pp.15t, 24b,
26, 27t. NHPA: pp.3, 6br, 11t. Oxford
Scientific Films: p.24t. Science Photo
Library: pp.9t, 13r, 46t, 48t, 51.

Special thanks go to: Dina Christy for
arranging studio photography.

Contents

INTRODUCTION   6

EXPLORING ALOE VERA   8

A HISTORY OF HEALING   10

ANATOMY OF ALOE VERA   14

ALOE VERA IN ACTION   16

ENERGY AND EMOTION   22
Flower essence   23

GROWING, HARVESTING,
AND PROCESSING   24

PREPARATIONS
FOR INTERNAL USE   28
Tonic drink   28
Detoxifying drink   29
Immune system fortifier   30
Daily power drink   31

PREPARATIONS
FOR EXTERNAL USE   32
Poultice   32
Lotion   33
Ointment   34
Moisturizing cream   35
Gargle/mouthwash   36
Douche   36
Eyewash   37
Nasal spray   37

NATURAL MEDICINE
FOR EVERYONE   38

HERBAL COMBINATIONS   40

HOW ALOE VERA WORKS   48

CONDITIONS CHART   52

GLOSSARY   56

FURTHER READING   58

USEFUL ADDRESSES   59

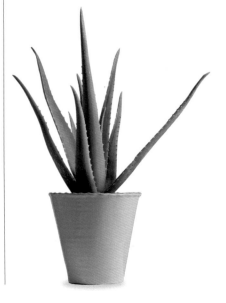

Introduction

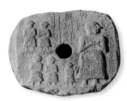

ABOVE *References to Aloe Vera first appeared on Sumerian clay tablets more than 3,000 years ago.*

ALOE VERA'S HISTORY *stretches back about 5,000 years. It is one of the most ancient medicinal plants, and the first written record of its use appears on a Sumerian clay tablet dated 1750* BCE. *Through the centuries and throughout the regions of the world in which it has been naturalized, Aloe Vera has been esteemed as a natural healer. It has been called "the miracle plant," "the medicine plant," and "the wand of heaven."*

Native to Africa, Aloe Vera is a perennial succulent plant with a thick, fibrous root. It produces a rosette of fleshy leaves that grow upward from its base, tapering to a point. Each thick leaf is edged with tiny spikes along its curving margins. Colors may vary from dull, bluish-gray to deep, bright green; a full-grown leaf can weigh 1–3lb (0.5–1.5kg). It is from the leaf that the soothing juice and translucent gel are extracted.

Aloe Vera is a xerophytic (drought-resistant) evergreen, which grows mainly in tropical

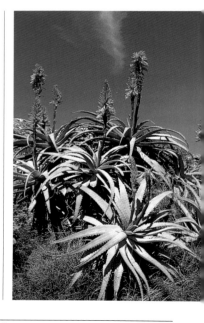

RIGHT *Mature Aloe Vera plants are a magnificent sight.*

BELOW *The succulent leaf of the cactuslike Aloe Vera plant.*

DEFINITION

Botanical family: *Liliaceae* – the lily family. Aloe Vera is related to onion, garlic, asparagus, and tulip.

Species: Aloe Vera's Latin name is also *Aloe vera. Vera* is Latin for "true," and the plant was given this name to differentiate it from other members of the aloe family and to identify it as the "healing aloe," although history and recent research shows that many Aloes share its healing qualities.

Other aloes

Aloe perryi, A. ferox, and *A. striatula* are some of the Aloe species that can be used in a similar way to Aloe Vera. *Aloe latifolia, A. saponaria,* and *A. tenuior,* all found in South Africa, are used primarily in the treatment of open wounds, worms, and parasitic skin infestations. *Aloe arborescens* has been cultivated for scientific use by the Russians.

and subtropical, desertlike savannas. Botanists classify it as xeroid, which means that if the leaves are cut, they can close off their cells to retain fluid. This makes them invaluable in the treatment of burns and wounds. It also means that the plant suffers no damage when a leaf is removed: it merely reseals itself.

IMPRESSIVE SIGHT

Often confused with the Agave, which it resembles, the Aloe Vera plant can reach the remarkable height of 60ft (20m), although generally they grow to about 4.5ft (1.5m). Each plant grows about 15 leaves, and blooms intermittently, producing stately erect spikes of drooping yellow, orange, or red tubular flowers on a woody stem.

FALSE CLAIMS

Aloe Vera has recently been hailed as a popular "cure-all." Many of the claims for its healing powers have been tried and tested over the centuries and substantiated by recent scientific research. However, some unjustifiable claims have been made, which is damaging because they result in increased skepticism among detractors. While Aloe Vera is an extremely useful medicinal herb, it is not a miracle cure-all, not least because both diet and lifestyle are also crucial to good health.

Exploring Aloe Vera

THERE ARE ABOUT *300 species in the genus Aloe, which grow in hot, arid climates around the world. The stiff, rugged, cactuslike appearance of Aloe Vera is as much a familiar sight in ornamental gardens and greenhouses as in those countries where the plant has become naturalized.*

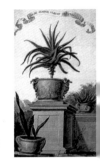

RIGHT *Aloe Vera is an attractive and hardy houseplant.*

WHERE TO FIND ALOE VERA

Although native to the dry, sunny areas of south and east Africa, Aloe Vera has also become naturalized in North Africa, the Middle East, the Mediterranean, the West Indies, Central and South America, Australia, the Far East, and parts of the United States and Russia. The Aloe Vera plant has also adapted well to greenhouse cultivation.

During the late 18th and early 19th centuries, Aloe Vera enjoyed a tremendous vogue among the wealthy collectors of exotic plants, and many important discoveries

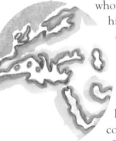

ABOVE *Aloe Vera grows in many parts of the world including Africa, the Middle and Far East, and Russia.*

about its properties were made during this period.

One of the most passionate collectors was the Prince Salm-Dyck (1773–1861), an amateur botanist from Germany, to whom much is owed for his meticulous observations of the Aloe Vera plant.

At one time Chatsworth House, in Derbyshire, housed the finest collection of Aloes in England. Today, the most impressive display is to be found at La Mortola, in Ventimiglia, Italy.

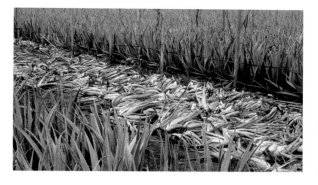

LEFT *Aloe Vera is grown commercially in areas of the world that have a warm, humid climate all year round.*

COMMERCIAL GROWERS

The largest area of Aloe Vera cultivation is the Rio Grande Valley of southern Texas. Here the excellent soil conditions – a mixture of clay, silt, and sand – and the warm, humid weather allow the plants to grow steadily throughout the year, which results in a high yield of nutrients. Commercial plantations can also be found in Mexico, the Caribbean, and Australia. Quality varies and, when you buy Aloe Vera, some people advise that you should look for the International Aloe Science Council (IASC) Seal of Approval. It is also wise to buy organic, nonpasteurized products for optimum healing results.

SOIL REQUIREMENTS

Being indigenous to the African savanna, Aloe Vera thrives best in a well-drained, gritty soil, with watering kept to a minimum. It needs plenty of heat and will not survive in temperatures that fall below 40°F (5°C). Most plants grown domestically in Northern Europe and parts of North America are best suited to container planting, which enables easy transportation from house to garden.

RIGHT *Potted Aloe Vera plants can be brought indoors when temperatures fall.*

A history of healing

ABOVE *Ancient texts have referred to the benefits of Aloe Vera.*

THE FIRST SERIOUS *writings on the therapeutic benefits of Aloe Vera are to be found in the Ebers Papyrus written around 1500* BCE *in which the Egyptians referred to the plant as* khet-awa, *meaning "the Plant of Immortality." For centuries Aloe Vera was used to heal wounds and burns. Its popularity waned briefly in the 19th century but it is now enjoying a renaissance.*

From the earliest times the reputation of Aloe Vera ensured its inclusion in any professional or domestic medicine chest. The ancient Egyptians recommended it for many ailments, particularly catarrh (see opposite). The Arabs called it "Desert Lily" and were probably the first to process the plant. Arab traders may have been responsible for the spread of Aloe Vera into Persia, India, and the Far East.

It is said that in 325 BCE, Alexander the Great was persuaded by his tutor, Aristotle, to seize the island of Socotra, in the Gulf of Aden, to obtain the Aloe Vera that grew there. Aristotle knew of the plant's

remarkable healing properties and that, because it could survive unplanted for several years, it could be carried as emergency treatment for wounds suffered by Alexander's army.

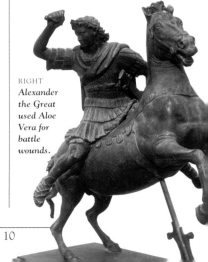

RIGHT *Alexander the Great used Aloe Vera for battle wounds.*

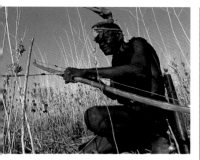

ABOVE *African hunters would rub their skin with Aloe Vera juice to mask their scent.*

In the first century CE, the Greek physician Dioscorides wrote in his *Materia Medica* that Aloe extract could be used to treat wounds, stomach complaints, constipation, hemorrhoids, headaches, "all griefs in the mouth," hair loss, insect bites, kidney ailments, and skin irritations.

WORLDWIDE USE

In its native Africa, the plant was traditionally taken to remedy stomachaches and guard against infection from insect bites. Hunters would rub Aloe Vera

RIGHT *Aloe Vera was used in ancient Egyptian remedies.*

juice on their skin to mask their scent so that they might approach their prey undetected.

The Chinese used Aloe Vera, but only in its resinous form – *Lu Hui* meaning "black deposit." The resin, which looked like small, dark chunks of amber, was not as potent as the growing plant but was respected for its power to heal skin. During the Sung dynasty (960–1276 CE), the resin was recommended for treating eczema.

In India during the fourth century BCE, people believed that Aloe Vera grew in the Garden of Eden. They called it *musabhar* (the silent healer) and used it to treat skin eruptions and inflammation.

EGYPTIAN REMEDY

The ancient Egyptians used Aloe Vera to relieve many ailments. The Coptic people, for example, treated a skin disease called psora with a mixture of Aloe Vera, baked cucumber, and wine. It was recorded that: "To expel catarrh in the nose take stibium, Aloe, dry myrrh, honey. Use it to annoint the nose for four days... Behold it is a true remedy."

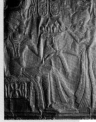

When the plant was introduced into the semitropical regions of the Americas, it thrived and was widely used by the peoples of those countries. In Mexico the juice was used to treat skin complaints and wounds and the sap was given as a purgative; in Central and South America, Aloe Vera was taken as a mild laxative. People also valued the juice as an effective insect repellent for both humans and animals.

ABOVE **Settlers brought Aloe Vera to the Americas.**

Paradoxically, Aloe Vera was sold on street markets of Latin America both to promote sleep and as an aphrodisiac.

GAINING POPULARITY

In the early Christian era, Aloe Vera featured in all advanced medical texts. Mass translations that became available in the 17th century encouraged the Jesuit priests of Spain to carry the plant, along with the Bible, to the New World.

ABOVE **Aloe Vera cream has a soothing effect on the skin.**

As Aloe Vera's popularity increased during the 18th century so did the competition to procure it; trade wars sprang up between rival countries – the Spanish, British, and Dutch in particular – to establish Aloe plantations in the New World.

By the 17th century, settlers in North America were using Aloe Vera to heal wounds and burns, a practice shared with many indigenous tribes. The Seminole people believed Aloe Vera had powers of rejuvenation and that a "Fountain of Youth" sprang from a pool within a cluster of Aloes.

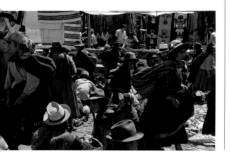

LEFT **Aloe Vera found its way into South America.**

19TH CENTURY DECLINE

Aloe Vera's popularity as a medicinal plant eventually waned, either because more easily obtainable remedies became available or because claims being made for the plant could not be substantiated. It is also quite likely that the gel was being adulterated and was therefore less effective. By the late 19th century, synthetic laboratory drugs had taken precedence over botanical compounds, and Aloe Vera fell completely from favor.

EARLY RESEARCH

Due to the urgent need during the 1930s to find a cure for radiation burns caused by experiments into X–ray techniques, the United States government started a program of research into the burn-healing properties of Aloe Vera. Successful experiments were carried out by Dr. E. E. Collins and his son Dr. Creston Collins, but because it was difficult to stabilize the juice and gel of Aloe Vera, their findings were considered inconclusive. Most research stopped until the 1960s

when improved techniques made stabilization possible, and public interest in Aloe Vera's therapeutic properties was once more aroused.

The Aloe is reputed to be one of the very few plants that is resilient enough to grow in areas where nuclear testing has taken place.

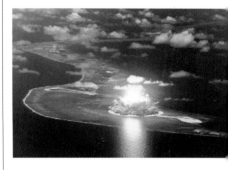

ABOVE *The hardy Aloe plant can even grow in nuclear testing sites.*

From the early 1950s, Russian scientists have carried out extensive research, but using the juice of *Aloe arborescens* rather than that of *Aloe vera*. They have investigated Aloe's use as a remedy for an impressive list of ailments, including eye disorders and bone tuberculosis as well as ear, nose, and throat conditions, and bronchial asthma.

Anatomy of Aloe Vera

THE WORD "ALOE" *comes from the Arabic word* alloeh, *which means "a bitter, shiny substance." This is an apt description for the dagger-shaped leaf, which has a bitter taste and spiky edges. These attributes are a deterrent to browsing animals and insects and may, in part, account for the plant's successful colonization.*

LEAVES

Beneath the inner surface of the leaf is a ridged lining that contains latex, or yellow sap. When dried and powdered, the sap is called "bitter aloes" and has long been used as a purgative. In the 17th century, Aloe Vera was grown for its sap in Barbados, thus gaining its other botanical name: *Aloe barbadensis*.

Within each leaf is clear, semi-liquid pulp, which botanists call parenchyma (tissue composed of soft, thin-walled cells). The pulp, which contains the gel, is removed in a "filleting" process. It is extracted with care to avoid contaminating it with bitter sap.

Aloe Vera juice is prepared commercially from the gel. The juice is usually taken internally, and the gel is applied to the skin. To be effective, the gel should not be diluted, and commercially prepared juice should contain at least 98 percent Aloe Vera juice.

LEFT *The large, dagger-shaped leaf is full of pulp.*

RIGHT *Gel and juice are sold in many forms.*

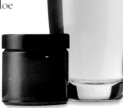

14

CHEMICAL CONSTITUENTS

It is the synergy (joint action) of the chemical constituents in Aloe Vera that makes it so effective in healing. It contains an amazing complexity of active compounds – 75 at the last count.

Constituents in the sap
Key constituents are barbaloin and isobarbaloin, which form "crystalline" aloin, "amorphous" aloin, aloe-emodin, resin, and volatile oil. These have strongly laxative effects. The purgative effects of aloin and aloe-emodin are powerful, so aloe sap in pills is combined with soothing herbs.

Constituents in the gel and juice
Small quantities of anthraquinones contribute to the gel's powerful anti-inflammatory and painkilling properties, helping to reduce swelling. The gel and juice contain a class of long-chain sugars known as mucopolysaccharides (MPS), normally found in all body cells. Production of MPS stops after the age of ten, so we then have to rely on outside sources; few plants are a

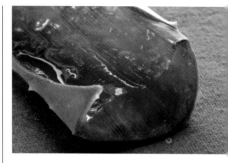

ABOVE *The key healing constituents can be found under the leaf's outer skin.*

richer source than Aloe Vera. It is thought that these sugars help boost the immune system, lubricate joints, and line the colon. Aloe Vera is especially rich in the MPS acemannan. Research has proved that acemannan stimulates the body's macrophages (see page 57) to produce interferon and interleukin, which stop viruses multiplying.

SHELF LIFE OF LEAVES
fresh leaves last for 2–3 months in the refrigerator, or up to 1 year in the freezer, either as they are or with the ends wrapped in plastic wrap; home dried or powdered leaves are not recommended.

Aloe Vera in action

KNOWN MAINLY AS *a remedy for skin conditions and constipation, Aloe Vera is also a natural detoxifier. The juice can be taken daily as a vegetable drink to cleanse the body, to build up resistance to infection, and to increase general energy levels and stamina.*

RIGHT *Aloe Vera is a natural detoxifier.*

HOW ALOE VERA CAN HELP

☀ Boosts the immune system and soothes and repairs damage to internal organs. Research is being carried out in this area to help improve the lives of people with AIDS and HIV.

☀ Boosts vitality and energy at those times when most needed. Athletes and students will find that because Aloe Vera both detoxifies and energizes, drinking the juice an hour before competitions or exams can give that extra surge of energy and concentration. However, it should be noted that too much juice drunk late in the evening will result in a sleepless night.

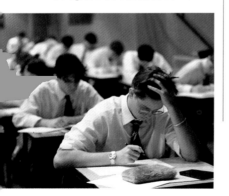

LEFT *Aloe Vera juice can give students the extra energy boost needed during examinations.*

Helps alleviate rheumatism and arthritis. Two tablespoons of juice in half a glass of water two to four times a day provides essential nutrients and noticeably improves arthritic and rheumatic conditions after two months or so. Massaging arthritic limbs with Aloe Vera cream improves circulation and reduces swelling.

Relieves eye, mouth, and vaginal infections.

Treats constipation; the anthraquinones in the sap are a potent laxative.

Helps alleviate a wide range of allergies, partly by reducing inflammatory reactions, thus controlling sneezing, wheezing, and indigestion.

Helps wounds to heal (and is currently being researched for possible use in cosmetic surgery).

Soothes stings and insect bites.

Soothes and heals burns,

RIGHT *Aloe Vera cream can be used to relief the pain of insect bites and bee stings.*

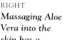

RIGHT
Massaging Aloe Vera into the skin has a soothing effect.

scalds, sunburn, cuts, and chapped skin (see page 18). Keeping a plant in the kitchen is recommended for emergency first aid.

Relieves skin conditions such as eczema and psoriasis.

HOW ALOE VERA AFFECTS THE BODY

Taken as a drink, Aloe Vera will cleanse and detoxify, and improve joint lubrication. This in turn will create more energy and improve mobility. In external injuries and swellings, sprains, and sunburn, the high water content of the gel (96%) carries nutrients to the site of the injury, improving cell regeneration. The anti-inflammatory and anesthetizing constituents reduce heat and pain.

ALOE VERA AND SUNBURN

For centuries Aloe Vera gel has been used to relieve burns. Although the risks of sunbathing are well publicized, many people still suffer from sunburn, even though the sun's ultraviolet-B rays can cause pain, premature skin aging, and skin cancer. Aloe Vera is not a sunblock, but it is a moisturizer, and will help reduce dehydration and burning. It is also anti-inflammatory.

"After-sun" lotions moisturize skin that is dry and damaged from wind and sun. Many of the products containing Aloe Vera have been developed in Australia and in southern parts of the United States, where sunburn is a serious risk all year round.

ABOVE *Aloe Vera is the basis for many skin-care products.*

The pure gel of Aloe Vera brings instant relief as it cools and anesthetizes. It also reduces irritation and, because it moisturizes, minimizes the risk of "peeling." The effects of mild sunstroke can be alleviated with a cooling application of cold Aloe Vera gel to the forehead and back of the neck.

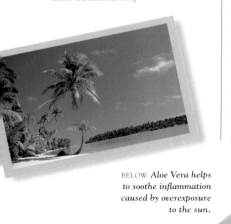

BELOW *Aloe Vera helps to soothe inflammation caused by overexposure to the sun.*

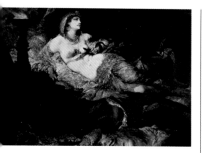

ABOVE *Throughout history,*
Aloe Vera has been used as a
beauty treatment.

REJUVENATING SKIN PREPARATION

Nefertiti and Cleopatra, two of history's most renowned beauties, were said to have bathed in Aloe Vera and had it made into lotions to enhance and preserve their beauty.

Ongoing research within the cosmetic industry indicates that the gel increases production of fibroblasts (cells in the dermis responsible for producing collagen, which keeps skin firm and supple). As we age, fibroblasts slow their collagen production, so the skin wrinkles more rapidly. Because Aloe Vera accelerates collagen production, facial lines become less pronounced.

Aloe Vera is especially effective as a moisturizer because it carries nutrients and moisture down through all layers of the skin. Its mucopolysaccharides (see page 15), which have moisture-binding properties, help Aloe Vera to protect the skin from moisture loss. Since it is nonallergenic and antibiotic, Aloe Vera is recommended for sensitive and problem skins. It is also reputed to remove age spots. It is always worth trying Aloe Vera gel on some skin disorders, because it is a natural antiseptic, antibiotic, and bactericide, the gel will inhibit the spread of infection. It also promotes rapid cell regeneration, helping blemishes to heal without scarring.

Scars from chickenpox and shingles can be minimized by applying Aloe Vera gel, and it can also help during the actual attack, cooling the associated heat and reducing itching. Internal use of the juice will also help treat the skin.

ABOVE *Aloe Vera is a prime first-aid treatment for burns.*

WHEN TO AVOID USING ALOE VERA

Generally Aloe Vera is a very safe plant to use. However, the latex or sap can be irritant and purgative, so it is removed during processing. Inferior brands of gel are sometimes made from poor grade Aloe Vera and may therefore be suspect, so look for the IASC Seal of Approval on the label (see page 9)..

❃ The yellow sap can be irritant – avoid contact with the skin.

❃ As with all herbal remedies, care should be taken not to exceed the recommended dose.

❃ Although Aloe Vera can alleviate the discomfort of hemorrhoids (piles), it can also exacerbate it, so use it with caution, especially if you are using it internally.

❃ Seek medical advice before taking Aloe Vera internally if you have a history of liver or gallbladder problems, cystitis, or uterine hemorrhage.

❃ Do not take internally during pregnancy or if breastfeeding because of laxative effects.

ALLERGY TEST

Although it is the safest of plants, there are a few people who are allergic to Aloe Vera. To find out if you are allergic, dab a small amount of juice or gel on the inside of your elbow. Leave for a few minutes. If there is a stinging sensation or a mild rash develops, wash the affected part and do not use Aloe Vera.

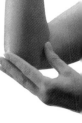

ABOVE *Testing for allergic reaction.*

USING ALOE VERA LEAVES

Cut a leaf as close to the main stem as possible and preferably from the base of the plant where the leaves are the oldest and the most potent. The plant will seal itself and suffer no damage.

RIGHT *Cutting an Aloe Vera leaf will not harm the plant.*

To use the leaf, wash it well and slice it in half lengthwise. Apply it as it is, gel side on the area to be treated, or remove the gel taking care to avoid the prickly skin. Some people prefer to let the gel drain into a container in order to avoid contamination from the yellow sap, which can be irritant. The sap will stay in the outer skin if it is not scraped.

To eat a little gel, peel off the outer leaf and wash off its yellow sap (this tastes bitter and may cause a mild stomach upset but it will do no lasting harm). The gel below this layer has a vaguely "plantish" but fairly neutral taste.

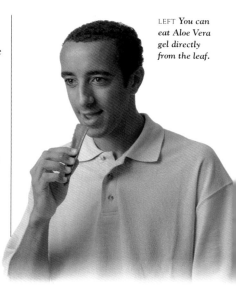

LEFT *You can eat Aloe Vera gel directly from the leaf.*

CASE STUDY: COLITIS

Rob had been suffering from pain in the lower stomach since he was 16 and had gradually been forced to eradicate all but the blandest foods from his diet. When he was 20 he spent a year working in Australia, where he was diagnosed as suffering from colitis. Despite treatment he continued to suffer severe pain and weight loss. Friends suggested he see a herbalist, who encouraged Rob to cut all wheat and dairy products from his diet and drink Slippery Elm "milk," made by whisking 1 tsp (5ml) of Slippery Elm powder into a glass of water, followed by 4 tsp (20ml) of Aloe Vera juice three times daily. Gradually Rob could eat a greater variety of food without discomfort and he gained a little weight. After a year he was fully recovered but continued a daily maintenance dose of Slippery Elm milk and 5 tsp (25ml) of Aloe Vera juice.

Although he was often traveling, Rob found it easy to maintain the daily dose while he was away because Aloe Vera is readily available without prescription.

Energy and emotion

ALOE VERA IS A *strong plant, symbolized by its power to survive hostile conditions including drought and even radiation, to regenerate itself, and on occasion to grow to heights that dwarf people. In those countries in which it grows abundantly, people consider it to be the "father of healing."*

ABOVE **The Aloe Vera flower is a symbol of strength and vigor.**

The appearance and feel of Aloe Vera gel fresh from the leaf is soothing and cooling, giving some indication of its ability to reduce inflammation and soothe burns. The sap is very bitter, and supports the function of both the stomach and liver, while restoring balance to the body as a whole. Bitter herbs work effectively on the small and large intestine, cleansing and strengthening, which in turn regulates the immune system. Conditions that might be termed "overheated" – high blood pressure, heart problems, constipation, inflammation, swellings – can be remedied by cooling, bitter herbs.

LEFT **Aloe Vera is soothing and cooling.**

ENERGY AND THE MIND

Aloe Vera energizes and invigorates, promoting a sense of well-being and promoting a more harmonious state between the emotions and the body, thus ensuring release of tension leading to an improvement in general health.

FLOWER REMEDIES

So dominant are the healing properties of the Aloe Vera leaf that little is known about the elegant spikes of flowers and what properties they might possess. They are associated with clarity and sharpness but there are no documented facts on their uses. However, if you would like to make a flower essence using Aloe Vera flowers, follow the method opposite.

PLANT SPIRIT ENERGIES

The plant's spirit embodies every part of the plant, not just the flowers. Aloe Vera can inhabit hostile environments. It protects itself from predators with its strong and sometimes piercing leaves, their unpalatable taste, and by constantly regenerating itself.

RIGHT *The plant helps to improve quality of life.*

Powerful and long-living, Aloe Vera shares these qualities with us without threat to its survival. It improves life for people who suffer from debilitating, chronic complaints that reduce energy.

TO MAKE A FLOWER ESSENCE

STANDARD QUANTITY

Approx. 1½ cups (350ml) each of spring water and brandy and 3–4 Aloe Vera flowers

1 *Submerge freshly picked Aloe Vera flowers in a shallow glass bowl containing spring water. Cover with a protective cloth of freshly washed white cheesecloth.*

2 *Leave the bowl in a quiet spot in the sunshine for three hours, or next to a window if you are indoors. Try to ensure that the flowers have at least three hours of continuous sun. If the flowers wilt sooner than this, remove them.*

3 *After three hours, use a twig to lift the flowers out of the bowl. Measure the amount of remaining liquid, and add an equal amount of brandy. Pour the mixture into sterilized, dark-glass bottles and label carefully.*

Recommended dosage

Adults: 4 drops under the tongue four times daily, or every half hour in times of crisis. Children: over 12 years, adult dose; 7–12 years, half adult dose; 1–7 years, quarter adult dose; younger than 1 year, smear the lips or tongue with Aloe flower water.

Growing, harvesting, and processing

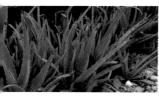

ALOE VERA HAS FEW *natural enemies but requires protection against frost and wind. However, if the conditions are suitable, it is a sturdy plant: it is not prone to disease, and it is pest-resistant. Conscientious Aloe Vera growers do not use chemical sprays, fertilizers, herbicides, or pesticides, preferring organic methods of cultivation. There have been successful experiments in growing Aloe Vera hydroponically (in a nutrient solution).*

ABOVE *Given the right conditions, Aloe Vera is a hardy pest-resistant plant.*

GROWING ALOE VERA

Commercial Cultivated on vast acreages, and grows well all year round. It propagates very rapidly, with new plants or "pups" growing from the root of the mother plant. These can be planted in open fields within nine months. Depending on weather and soil conditions, a plant will reach maturity in three to five years.

LEFT *Aloe Vera is grown commercially on huge plantations.*

Aloe vera is cultivated in well-drained, gritty soil that is a mixture of clay, silt, and sand. The weather must be warm and humid, never below 40°F (5°C).

Three or four species of Aloe are cultivated commercially, but only A. *vera* (also known as A. *barbadensis*) is used for healing.

Homegrown Although it is possible to grow Aloe Vera from seed, this is a long and not entirely foolproof exercise. Many nurseries sell Aloe Vera plants, and it is best to buy a sturdy plant that is at least 18 months old because it takes the leaves two to three years to reach their full medicinal potential. Alternatively, obtain a rooted offshoot from a friend and bring it to maturity.

Aloe Vera is fairly hardy, but it is indigenous to temperate and subtropical zones so it should be kept indoors unless temperatures are quite high. The plants need plenty of space, so plant in dry, gritty soil in a fairly large pot with adequate drainage. They need repotting when they send out new shoots. If the shoots are left with the mother plant none will thrive, but wait until shoots grow to 2in (5cm) high before transplanting. Water well, then abstain for three weeks, which will force each shoot to produce extra roots, thus ensuring more robust plants.

Aloe Vera plants grow slowly and need little watering, so wait until the soil feels dry before adding a cup or two of water.

ABOVE *Aloe Vera are robust plants that need little watering.*

If the soil becomes excessively dry in hot weather, stand the pot in water until the soil is only just moist, making sure it is well drained when removed. If possible, use rain or purified water because Aloe Vera is sensitive to fluoride – this may cause brown spotting on the leaves, which in turn may harm its biochemistry.

Aloe Vera plants enjoy warmth, but direct sunlight on their leaves may turn them brown. However, insufficient light will make the leaves droop and flatten. Lack of water results in inward-curling leaves, and bruising causes leaves to have brown marks and dried edges. Any of these problems may occur if the plant is placed too close to a radiator or other direct source of heat.

The bitter taste of Aloes will keep the house and any plants growing near them free from insects.

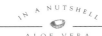
HARVESTING

Commercial Leaves are ready for harvesting when they weigh 1–1½lb (450–700g) each and measure about 1½in (3cm) at the base of the 2ft (60cm) leaf. The whole process of harvesting is done by hand, making it highly labor-intensive. The majority of Aloe Vera products come from companies who have a massive production level and total control over the process, from planting through to harvesting and processing.

When harvested, only two or three leaves are removed from the base of the plant at a time and cut at a point high enough to ensure that the young inner leaves are not damaged and can go on to produce the next year's harvest.

Homegrown There is no specific time for harvesting Aloe Vera. Provided that the plant is sturdy and of sufficient age, a leaf can be removed whenever the need arises. However, it is best not to start cutting leaves until the plant is about three years old.

When cutting a leaf, take care to cut it close to the stem to ensure that it will reseal itself, and choose an older leaf at the bottom of the plant because it will be more medicinally potent. This will also maintain the handsome appearance of the Aloe Vera plant.

BELOW *Aloe Vera plants are cultivated commercially on a massive level.*

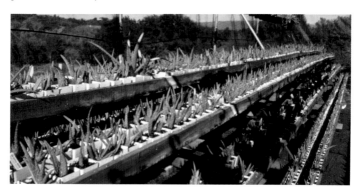

PROCESSING

Commercial In the summer, processing takes place on the same day as harvesting, but in cooler months it may occur up to 24 hours later.

Leaves are taken to conveyor belts where they are washed and the tops and bottoms removed. Then the leaf is "filleted" – cut lengthwise and the outside rind removed to reveal the gel. This is usually done by hand to avoid damaging the leaf and to make sure the sap-containing channels beneath the skin are not punctured. If this happens, the gel will be contaminated with bitter, purgative sap. The rind is used as organic fertilizer, while the jellylike pulp is ground to a near-liquid state and piped into stainless steel vats for processing. Hand filleting is expensive, but machine processing could allow impurities into the gel.

The last step is stabilization, which inhibits oxidization of the gel and preserves nutrients. This

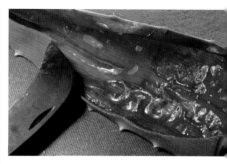

ABOVE *Filleting is usually done by hand.*

ABOVE *The top and bottom are removed before the leaf is filleted.*

does not interfere with the plant's healing properties but does ensure that the gel retains its freshness. All Aloe Vera products contain a preservative. Some are pasteurized, but this heating process is thought by many to destroy valuable enzymes and change the protein structure. Several companies use a heat-free process, which does not cause chemical reactions.

Homegrown Leaves are sealed in plastic wrap and refrigerated for up to three weeks, or frozen for three months, and then filleted.

Preparations for internal use

NOWADAYS, *commercially prepared Aloe Vera juice, gel, and powder are pure, long-lasting, and convenient to use. It is possible to buy Aloe Vera in capsules, in specially formulated laxative pills, and in a range of products to improve health and treat ailments.*

ABOVE **Aloe Vera is available in capsule form.**

MORNING TONIC DRINK

This drink is best consumed fresh to ensure the maximum nutritional benefits. However, you can make the vegetable juice in advance without adding the Aloe Vera juice and seasoning and keep it in a refrigerator for up to eight hours. Before serving, return the vegetable juice to the food processor and blend in the Aloe Vera juice, then season to taste.

RIGHT **Spinach can be acidic and bell peppers can cause wind if used in excess.**

TO MAKE A TONIC DRINK

MAKES 4 GLASSES

6oz (175g) fresh, green raw vegetables
4oz (115g) carrots, peeled and chopped
4oz (115g) bell peppers, skinned, deseeded, and chopped
4oz (115g) tomatoes, skinned and chopped
salt and freshly ground black pepper
4 tbsp Aloe Vera juice

1 *Wash, trim, and chop the green vegetables. Put into a food processor with the other vegetables. Blend until smooth and season to taste. Refrigerate for up to 3 days.*

2 *Before drinking, stir in the Aloe Vera juice.*

Recommended dosage
See page 29.

DETOXIFYING DRINK

This easy-to-prepare drink is best consumed fresh. Lemon juice is a tremendous cleanser and detoxifier, clearing the stomach of excess acid, scouring the blood, and cooling and clearing the skin. Apple and Aloe Vera also cleanse and detoxify. All three ingredients are rich in antioxidants, which fight infection. This drink relieves allergies and skin problems, and treats constipation. It also boosts the immune system.

Buy freshly squeezed apple juice (not made from a concentrate) or make your own, in which case the seeds will be included and their pectin, which has detoxifying properties. To make the apple juice, wash and chop six medium-size eating apples (no need to peel or core) and feed into the juicer. Collect the juice.

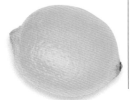

BOVE AND
IGHT **Apple and
emon juice are
oth effective in
leansing and
etoxify the body.**

TO MAKE A DETOXIFYING DRINK

MAKES 1 GLASS

10fl oz (300ml) apple juice
2fl oz (50ml) Aloe Vera juice
freshly squeezed juice
of ¼ to 1 lemon

1 *Pour the apple juice
into a pitcher, then
quickly pour in the
Aloe Vera juice.*

2 *Add the lemon
juice to taste
and stir well.
Consume
immediately.*

Recommended dosage

*Adults: 1 glass one to three times
daily. If pregnant or breastfeeding,
remember the juice will have a
laxative effect, so
use it with care.
Children: 7 years
and over, adult
dose; 3–7 years,
half adult dose;
1–3 years, 20
drops morning and
evening; younger
than 1 year,
10 drops daily.*

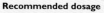

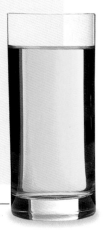

IMMUNE SYSTEM FORTIFIER

This drink strengthens and supports the immune system, helping the body to fight coughs, colds, and other infections. It has no components that could overexert the immune system and works purely as a supportive tonic, used for thousands of years in China. Aloe Vera's polysaccharide constituents stimulate the immune system, so this combination has a very balancing and beneficial effect.

The Reishi mushroom, which is widely available as a powder, is renowned for its fortifying support to the immune system. It is sometimes known by its Latin name, *Ganoderma lucidum*.

ABOVE **Reishi mushroom powder.**

Organic red grape juice, which you can buy or make, flavors the drink and is rich in powerful antioxidants and other constituents that help the immune system to fight infections. This drink should be drunk immediately or within eight hours.

TO MAKE AN IMMUNE SYSTEM FORTIFIER

MAKES 2–3 GLASSES

2fl oz (50ml) Aloe Vera juice
3 cups (750ml) organic red grape juice
2 tsp Reishi mushroom powder

1 Combine the Aloe Vera and red grape juice in a pitcher.

2 Whisk in the Reishi mushroom powder, then pour into a glass and drink before the powder settles at the bottom. If you prefer to sip it, stir occasionally.

Recommended dosage

Adults: Up to 6 glasses daily. It can be beneficial if pregnant or breast-feeding, but if mother's or baby's stools become too loose, stop immediately.
Children: over 12 years, adult dose; 7–12 years, half adult dose; 3–7 years, quarter adult dose; younger than 3 years, 3 tsp (15ml) daily.

DAILY POWER DRINK

Aloe Vera juice added to a Superfood drink (available from health stores, see page 59) is a powerful addition to meals, providing extra energy without increasing calorific intake. It can replace up to one meal a day for a month if you want to regulate your weight but still receive adequate nutrients. It will keep for eight hours in the refrigerator.

Aloe Vera aids the digestive process by ensuring nutrients are broken down and assimilated.

Superfood contains organic plant ingredients, which deliver a wide range of body builders. Some plant components act like natural RNA and DNA, reading the body's "blueprint" and helping regenerate healthy tissue, while others help create vital body hormones or help detoxify the body. Superfood is rich in non-essential fatty acids, vitamins, minerals, pectins, trace elements, essential oils, and organic acids.

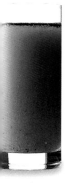

ABOVE *A power drink is full of nutrients.*

TO MAKE A DAILY POWER DRINK

MAKES ONE LARGE GLASS

freshly squeezed juice of 1 lemon
2 tbsp (30ml) Superfood
2½ cups (700ml) organic fruit juice,
(or use half fruit juice and half spring water)
2fl oz (50ml) Aloe Vera juice

1 *Put all the ingredients in a blender or food processor and process until thoroughly blended.*

2 *Pour into a large glass and drink immediately.*

Recommended dosage

Adults: One large glass daily, or double dose if convalescing or body building. If pregnant or breastfeeding, take only 3 tsp (15ml) daily for three days, then increase the dose slowly until it suits mother and baby.

Children: over 12 years, adult dose; 7–12 years, half adult dose; 3–7 years, quarter adult dose; younger than 3 years, 3 tsp (15ml) daily.

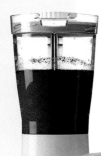

Preparations for external use

Aloe Vera gel is an outstanding herbal remedy for skin conditions. You can apply it on its own or use it in poultices, ointments, lotions, and creams to soothe, heal, and moisturize.

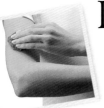

ABOVE **Aloe Vera is used to treat a variety of skin conditions.**

ABOVE **A poultice of healing herbs ensure deep penetration into a sore.**

POULTICE FOR BURNS, LEG ULCERS, AND BEDSORES

A poultice is often the best way of ensuring that healing herbs penetrate deep into a sore. Marshmallow, Comfrey, and Aloe Vera speed healing and are valuable in the treatment of burns, leg ulcers, or bedsores. Powdered Slippery Elm protects the skin and adds substance to the mixture.

CAUTION

Always seek medical advice for a severe burn, ulcer, or bedsore to ensure that infection does not arise and any shock is dealt with professionally.

RIGHT **Poultice of herbs, Aloe Vera gel, and oil.**

TO MAKE A POULTICE

STANDARD QUANTITY

1 part each powdered Marshmallow root and Comfrey root
1½ parts powdered Slippery Elm bark
Aloe Vera gel, and olive oil or any suitable pure vegetable oil (enough to make a paste – see below)

1 *Put the herbs in a bowl. Using ¾ Aloe Vera gel to ¼ olive oil, add enough to create a pliable paste. As a guide, for 1½oz (40g) of powder you will need 2fl oz (50ml) of Aloe gel and olive oil.*

2 *Coat the affected area with a thin layer of olive oil, and cover with a pastry-thick layer of paste. Cover with clean cheesecloth, secure with plastic wrap, and leave on for 24 hours. Reapply every 24 hours until the burn or ulcer is healed.*

SOOTHING LOTION

This soothing lotion is ideal for relieving sunburn or to keep in the kitchen as a first-aid remedy for minor burns and scalds (but first immerse the affected part in cold water for ten minutes.) Aloe Vera gel is soothing, cooling, and helps the skin to regenerate; St. John's Wort cold-pressed oil is antiseptic, soothing, and anti-inflammatory.

TO MAKE A LOTION

STANDARD QUANTITY

For the St. John's Wort oil, use enough chopped fresh St. John's Wort flowers and top leaves to fill a clean 2fl oz (50ml) glass jar, plus 3 tbsp (45ml) cold-pressed, extra-virgin olive oil (or buy St. John's Wort cold-pressed oil and continue from step 5) 1fl oz (30ml) Aloe Vera gel

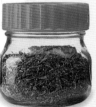

1 Put some St. John's Wort buds, flowers, and a few top leaves in the jar so that it is three-quarters full. Pack the herb tightly to make a stronger, more concentrated oil.

2 Add sufficient olive oil to cover the herb, secure the lid, and shake well. Don't let the herbs oxidize (turn brown) by letting them protrude above the oil. Shaking the jar frequently will help the herb to settle below the oil's surface.

3 Place the jar in a warm, sunny position. Leave for at least two weeks, although there is no strict time limit on the "warming phase."

You can leave it for three months provided you shake the jar daily.

4 Strain the mixture through a jelly bag or wine press. If using a jelly bag, leave it overnight, then thoroughly squeeze any remaining oil from the bag.

5 To make the lotion, mix 2fl oz (50ml) of the oil with the Aloe Vera gel. Transfer it to a sterilized dark glass jar, label, and store in a refrigerator for up to three months.

Recommended usage
Adults and children: apply liberally, as often as required.

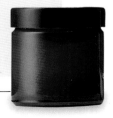

OINTMENTS AND CREAMS

Making your own ointments and creams can ensure that they are specifically suited to your own health needs and will provide quick and easy remedies for a wide range of external problems.

ALOE VERA OINTMENT

Gently massaging swollen joints, aching muscles, and varicose veins with this soothing, easily absorbed ointment reduces inflammation and swelling. It is also useful for cuts, burns, and some dry skin infections. Massage it into the affected part regularly.

TO MAKE AN OINTMENT

STANDARD QUANTITY

approx. 12 tsp (60g) coconut butter or beeswax (you may need to add more in a warm climate or less in a cold climate), 2fl oz (60ml) coconut oil, 4fl oz (120ml) olive oil, 1 cup (250ml) Aloe Vera juice

TIP

You can use Aloe Vera juice as an antiperspirant. Just put some juice into an atomizer, keep it refrigerated for up to three months and use as required.

1 *Melt the coconut butter or beeswax and oils in a heatproof bowl over a pan of hot water on the stove.*

2 *Remove the bowl from the heat and slowly pour the Aloe Vera gel into the wax* mixture, beating it constantly until the mixture is cold.

3 *Pour the ointment into a sterilized dark glass jar, seal, and label. If refrigerated, the ointment may further solidify but will melt at room temperature. It will keep for two years.*

Recommended usage
Adults and children: Apply liberally and as often as required.

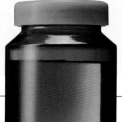

RIGHT *Soothing Aloe Vera ointment is easily absorbed into the skin.*

ALOE VERA MOISTURIZING CREAM

Here is a gentle moisturizing cream that, when used over a period of time, will improve the quality of the skin, eradicate small scars and age spots, and smooth out facial lines.

TO MAKE A MOISTURIZING CREAM

STANDARD QUANTITY

1 tbsp (15ml) beeswax, 6 tbsp (90ml) almond oil,
¼ tsp (1ml) borax, 3 tbsp (45ml) spring or distilled water,
2 tbsp (30ml) Aloe Vera juice, 1 capsule each vitamins A and E

1 *Place the beeswax and oil together in a heatproof bowl and heat over a double saucepan of hot water.*

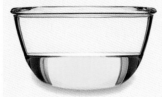

TIP

You can use Aloe Vera juice as a facial toner before applying moisturizer.

2 *Dissolve the borax in the spring water in another bowl by heating in the same way. Warm the Aloe Vera juice in a separate bowl.*

3 *When the beeswax has melted, remove all bowls from the heat. Mix the borax and water mixture with the Aloe Vera juice and pour slowly into the beeswax mixture, beating constantly until the mixture begins to cool.*

4 *Prick the vitamin capsules and beat the contents into the mix. Continue beating until cold.*

5 *When the mixture is cold, transfer it to a sterilized dark glass pot, seal, and label carefully.*

Recommended usage

Adults and children: Apply the cream liberally and as often as required.

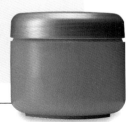

ALOE VERA DOUCHE

This douche is useful for all types of vaginal infections: candida, thrush, and other more chronic, persistent problems. Aloe Vera juice will soothe and heal vaginal mucous membranes and promote a positive immune system reaction in the area.

ALOE AND OAK GARGLE AND MOUTHWASH

This mouthwash is ideal for any infection, soreness, or inflammation of the throat, gums, or mouth, including mouth ulcers and gum disease. Oak is astringent; Aloe Vera is anti-inflammatory and soothing; both are antiseptic.

TO MAKE A VAGINAL DOUCHE

STANDARD QUANTITY

2 cups (500ml) undiluted Aloe Vera juice

1 *Strain the Aloe Vera juice through a colander or sieve lined with clean cheesecloth. Normally this is unnecessary, but any little pieces will clog the douche. Use as normal for a douche, following the instructions that come with a douche kit. (Douche kits are available from some health food stores as well as pharmacies.)*

TO MAKE A GARGLE/MOUTHWASH

STANDARD QUANTITY

2fl oz (50ml) spring water, 2fl oz (50ml) Aloe Vera juice, 2fl oz (50ml) Oak bark, twig or leaf tincture, 1 tsp (5ml) fine sea salt

1 *Put all the ingredients in a sterilized bottle. Screw on the lid and shake well, so that all the salt eventually dissolves. Store in a refrigerator for up to three weeks.*

Recommended usage

Adults: Use up to four times daily. Children: adult dose (swallowing small amounts is not harmful); unsuitable for younger than 1 year.

ALOE VERA EYEWASH

This eyewash is useful for sore eyes and conjunctivitis. Add a minute pinch of salt to each eye bath to help prevent the leaching of minerals from the eyes.

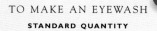

ALOE VERA NASAL SPRAY

Aloe Vera nasal spray is useful for nasal polyps, colds, and allergies. Goldenseal disinfects and reduces inflammation. You can buy empty pump sprays from pharmacies.

TO MAKE AN EYEWASH

STANDARD QUANTITY

2 tsp (10ml) Aloe Vera juice and
2 tsp (10ml) spring or distilled water

1 *Pour the Aloe Vera juice and distilled water into a clean glass and stir together well.*

Recommended usage

Apply a few drops to the eye, blinking continuously. Treat both eyes to prevent the infection from spreading. Sterilize the eye bath before using on the other eye. Adults, and children over 3 years, can use the eyewash up to three times daily, for 2–3 weeks. For children younger than 3 years, consult a doctor or qualified herbalist.

TO MAKE A NASAL SPRAY

STANDARD QUANTITY

4 tsp (20ml) spring or distilled water
6 tsp (30ml) Aloe Vera juice
2 tsp (10ml) Goldenseal tincture

1 *Pour all the ingredients into a clean glass and stir well.*

2 *Transfer the mixture to an empty pump spray. Store in the refrigerator for up to six months.*

Recommended usage

Tilt the head back and spray into each nostril. Adults: use the spray on each nostril up to five times daily. Children: over 12 years, adult dose; 7–12 years, half adult dose; 3–7 years, quarter adult dose; younger than 3 years, consult a doctor or qualified herbalist.

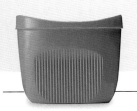
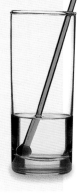

Natural medicine for everyone

FOR CENTURIES *Aloe vera has been a great and gentle healer and is believed to be safe for most people, even those members of society who might be considered the most vulnerable, such as invalids, pregnant women, children, and the elderly.*

ABOVE *Aloe Vera remedies can be used by people of all ages.*

PREGNANCY

In the past it was considered to be unwise for pregnant women to take Aloe Vera internally because it caused bowel spasm. However, this was mainly due to the use of inferior brands in which aloin (the purgative substance in the sap) had contaminated the gel. A pure gel will not have this effect, so check the label for the IASC Seal of Approval (see page 9).

Many pregnant women take Aloe Vera as a tonic because it increases energy levels, improves digestion, and minimizes heartburn, morning sickness, and constipation. Folic acid, which is useful to pregnant women because it helps iron assimilation (see page 56) is also present in Aloe Vera. However, it may not be advisable for nursing mothers to take Aloe Vera in case the baby's stools become too loose. But for a constipated baby, this would be an ideal choice.

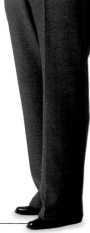

RIGHT *Good-quality Aloe Vera is even safe for pregnant women.*

CHILDREN

Children may benefit from Aloe Vera in several ways.

🌿 Applied to external injuries, it is gentle and effective, and heals without scarring; the novelty of using it straight from the leaf may be a distraction from pain.

🌿 It is a gentle, nonhabit-forming treatment for constipation, while it may also, paradoxically, dispel minor bouts of diarrhea.

🌿 Older children and teenagers, particularly those undergoing the stress of examinations or competitions, will benefit from an Aloe Vera drink an hour or so before the event. This will give a boost of energy and concentration.

🌿 It can help children who suffer from allergies. It helps to improve the immune system, gut, and inflammatory responses.

> **CAUTION**
>
> Do not give Aloe vera to children at night because it energizes and may therefore result in sleeplessness.

ELDERLY PEOPLE

Some of the progressive conditions associated with aging may be inhibited by the persistent use of Aloe Vera.

🌿 Arthritic and rheumatic conditions are noticeably improved by drinking the juice and massaging with the cream.

🌿 Aloe Vera helps in the treatment of many ailments associated with aging: high blood pressure, heart conditions, diabetes, as well as bowel, liver, kidney, and digestive disorders.

🌿 Aloe Vera juice energizes, and the gel improves skin and hair.

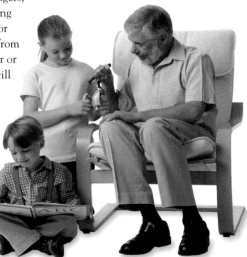

RIGHT *Aloe Vera is suitable for the young and elderly alike.*

Herbal combinations

HERBAL COMBINATIONS *are used where the effect of a single herb needs to be helped in a particular way. If you are pregnant, breast-feeding, or have a serious medical condition, you must consult your doctor or a qualified medical herbalist first in case some herbs are contraindicated.*

LEFT *Aloe Vera can help ease allergies caused by animals or pollen.*

ALLERGIES

This tincture or tea will ease the discomfort of hay fever, mucus buildups in sinuses and lungs, and irritated eyes.

Tincture formula 2fl oz (50ml) Aloe Vera juice, 4 tsp (20ml) each of Plantain leaf, Nettle root, and Elderflower tincture.

Dosage Adults: 1 tsp (5ml) four times a day. Children: over 12 years, adult dose; 7–12 years, half adult dose; 3–7 years, quarter adult dose; younger than 3 years, 3 drops twice daily.

Tea formula 5fl oz (150ml) Aloe Vera juice, 7fl oz (200ml) each of Plantain leaf, Nettle root, and Elderflower tea.

Dosage Adults: 3 cups (750ml) daily. Children: over 12 years, adult dose; 7–12 years, half adult dose; 3–7 years, a quarter adult dose; younger than 3 years, 2 tsp (10ml) twice daily.

Aloe Vera mobilizes the immune system and soothes inflamed tissues.

Plantain is rich in antihistamines and reduces the inflammation associated with allergies. It also reduces excessive mucus and soothes mucous membranes.

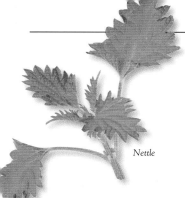

Nettle

Elderflower is renowned for soothing coughs and allergies. It helps tone impaired linings of the nose and throat and increases their resistance to pollen, dust, and infection.

Nettle relieves breathing problems created by allergic reactions and is especially helpful for allergic rhinitis, hay fever, asthma, and itchy skin conditions because of its antiallergenic, tonic, and astringent constituents.

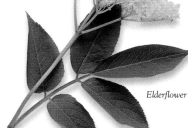

Elderflower

CASE STUDY: ARTHRITIS

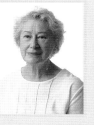

Margie Dean, a retired secretary in her 60s, found that, as a result of her work, her neck and fingers were becoming very stiff with arthritis. Her physiotherapist gave her a series of exercises to promote flexibility and suggested that she try Aloe Vera.

At the time, Margie could barely turn her head, and her fingers were curled to the extent that she could not pick up a knife and fork. She agreed to take 4 tsp (20ml) Aloe Vera juice four times daily.

She also applied the gel, cold from the refrigerator, to her hands and neck and massaged a cream gently into the painful areas. The worst of the pain began to ease almost immediately and after two months she started to experience the full benefits. Now she can turn her head easily from side to side and pick up a pen without difficulty. Margie has reduced her Aloe Vera intake to a maintenance dose of 4 tsp (20ml) twice a day. She has also improved some aspects of her diet.

BURNS

This spray combines instant cooling action with herbs that soothe burns. Using a spray means the actual burn need not be touched. Always run cold water on a burn for ten minutes. If serious, contact your doctor or call an ambulance.

Formula 2 cups (500ml) Aloe Vera juice, 8 drops organic Lavender essential oil, 1 cup (250ml) Witchhazel water. Mix the ingredients together, and put into a spray atomizer. Label and store in a refrigerator for up to six months.

Usage Spray directly on the burn, reapplying when pain returns.

Aloe Vera contains allantoin, which promotes rapid cell division, creating rapid skin regrowth. It naturally soothes and helps to diminish the heat and inflammation of burns. Lavender is the only essential oil that is beneficial for burns when used neat. It soothes, cools, and accelerates healing while preventing infection.

The Witchhazel water soothes and heals, complementing the other two herbs.

Comfrey root

Aloe Vera oil in capsules

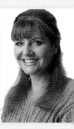

Comfrey powder

CASE STUDY: BURNS

While deep-frying some food, Janet let the fat boil over and run into the gas flame below. In an attempt to smother the flames, her hands were burned. Janet's neighbor, Karen, who was with her at the time, put Janet's hands under cold running water for ten minutes, then cut a leaf from her Aloe Vera plant, cut it lengthwise, and gave immediate first aid by laying it, gel-side down, on Janet's hands. She then bandaged the gel into place. The burns were painful but minor, and Karen instructed Janet to keep the bandage on overnight and replace it in the morning if necessary.

The next day Janet was amazed to find that not only had the pain stopped completely but the skin was cool and there was no break or blistering. She applied gel from a second leaf and later switched to commercially produced Aloe Vera gel and then also Calendula oil to continue the speedy healing process.

LEFT *Aloe Vera spray can help soothe and cool painful burns.*

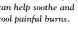

GENTLE COLON CLEANSING FORMULA

A safe way to ease the discomfort of constipation, this formula is suitable for the young and old alike. It contains herbs that are gentle, powerful, and nonhabit-forming.

CAUTION

Before taking this colon formula, consult a herbalist if you are pregnant, breastfeeding, or if you have hemorrhoids.

Formula 2 tbsp powdered, dried Psyllium husks, 1 tsp (5ml) Yellow Dock root tincture, 2fl oz (50ml) Aloe Vera juice, and spring water or fruit juice (optional, as needed).

Put the Psyllium husks in a glass and add the fluids, including a little water or fruit juice to taste. Stir and drink immediately. If you allow it to stand, the husks will expand in the glass instead of in the colon and the mixture will have to be eaten like a pudding.

Dosage Adults: Total quantity of formula twice daily. Children: over 12 years, adult dose; 7–12 years, half adult dose? 3–7 years, quarter adult dose; younger than 3 years, consult an herbalist.

Yellow Dock root

Psyllium husks expand in the bowel, becoming gelatinous. They soothe any irritation and inflammation, and they ease the passage of stools through the colon by making them bulkier and softer.

Yellow Dock improves bile flow, which is vital for bowel performance; its anthroquinone content acts as a gentle laxative and cleanser.

Psyllium husks

Aloe Vera has the same properties as Yellow Dock. It soothes and helps repair any bowel tissue damage caused by persistent constipation.

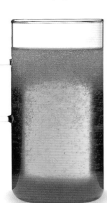

LEFT **An Aloe Vera colon cleansing drink.**

"LEAKY GUT" FORMULA

Complementary practitioners believe that, as a result of allergies and digestive conditions including Candida (yeast overgrowth in the gut), the intestines can become inflamed and hyperpermeable. They leak, behaving more like a "colander" than a secure "bowl," allowing toxic substances to be released into the body. This results in rashes and other allergic reactions.

Formula 1 tsp (5ml) Echinacea root tincture, 1 tsp (5ml) Artichoke leaf tincture, 1 tsp (5ml) Barberry root tincture, 2 tsp (10ml) Meadowsweet flower and leaf tincture, 1 tsp (5ml) Aloe Vera leaf juice, 1 probiotic capsule (or equivalent powder – it must contain acid stable, human compatible, bacteria).

Put the four tinctures into a sterilized container. If you wish to avoid the small amount of alcohol contained in the tinctures, add a few drops of boiling water to the

Echinacea root

container, which will evaporate 98.5% of the alcohol in five minutes. When cool, add the Aloe Vera juice and probiotic powder (or take a probiotic capsule independently).

Dosage Adults: 2 tsp (10ml) twice daily. Children: over 12 years, adult dose; 7–12 years, half adult dose; 3–7 years, quarter adult dose; unsuitable for children younger than 3 years.

Echinacea supports the immune and digestive systems, which is vital for a gut that is overwhelmed

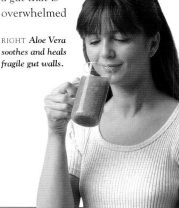

RIGHT *Aloe Vera soothes and heals fragile gut walls.*

by harmful fungi and bacteria.

Artichoke tones the digestive system. Its strongly bitter substances increase saliva flow and the production of pancreatic and stomach juices.

Barberry contains berberine and hydrastine, which have an antimicrobial action, and the herb also supports the digestive system, including the liver.

Meadowsweet promotes the regrowth of healthy stomach tissue and balances digestive juice production.

Aloe Vera is first class at soothing inflammation, supporting the immune system, and healing fragile gut walls. It also assists digestion, partly by promoting growth of "good" gut bacteria.

The probiotic capsule is an important part of the formula. The gut normally contains plenty of "good" bacteria that can assist with digestion, but in someone who has Candida, these bacteria are overwhelmed by harmful microorganisms. The probiotic powder helps restore normal balance of bacteria in the intestines.

Aloe Vera leaf

barberry bark

Meadowsweet

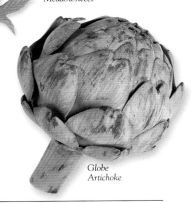

Globe Artichoke

CAUTION

Do not take this formula if you are pregnant or breastfeeding.
Consult a qualified medical herbalist before using Echinacea if you have cancer, HIV, or an autoimmune disease such as rheumatoid arthritis.

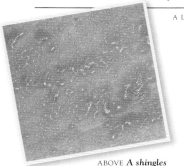

ABOVE *A shingles rash is very painful.*

SHINGLES

Few lotions and creams are able to relieve the severe itching caused by shingles, and many simply make the inflammation and pain worse. However, this gel formula should help to ease the discomfort.

Formula Use 1 part each of Aloe Vera gel, Witchhazel gel, and St. John's Wort cold-pressed oil. Mix together a squirt each in the palm of the hand and apply to the rash, or mix in a dish and apply with absorbent cotton. Let dry before replacing clothing. By mixing this formula in the hand, however, the whole operation is quick and simple, especially if self-administered.

RIGHT *Shingles are soothed with an Aloe Vera formula.*

Usage Adults: apply up to five times daily.

Both gels cool and soothe, helping to reduce pain, itchiness, and inflammation. The Aloe Vera helps the immune system to fight the *herpes zoster* virus that is causing the rash.

The same can be said of St. John's Wort oil, which has antiviral qualities; it is also anti-inflammatory and healing.

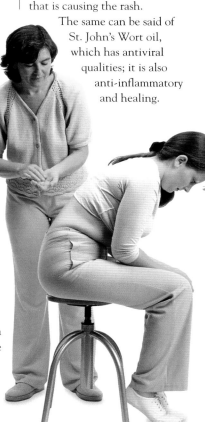

CHINESE IMMUNE SYSTEM TONIC

This formula is very useful in the treatment of conditions that impair the immune system, such as postviral fatigue syndrome and mononucleosis. It is also excellent for convalescents.

Schisandra

Formula 2 tsp (10ml) Astragalus root tincture, 2 tsp (10ml) Rehmannia root tincture, 2 tsp (10ml) Schisandra berry tincture, 6 tsp (30ml) Aloe Vera juice.

Mix the tinctures together. (This can be done in advance.) Just before you take the dose, add the Aloe Vera juice. In this way the formula will remain fresh.

Dosage Adults: 1–2 tsp (5–10ml) two, but preferably four, times daily. Children: over 12 years, adult dose; 7–12 years, half adult dose; under 7 years, consult a doctor or a qualified herbalist.

Astragalus, Rehmannia, and Schisandra – all tonic herbs in Traditional Chinese Medicine – are increasingly being used in Western herbalism. They all support and stimulate the entire body in a very balanced and regenerative way and nourish the immune system so that it can work efficiently without becoming exhausted.

Aloe Vera is rich in mucopolysaccharides, which maintain the immune system (see page 15), and anthroquinones, which have an antimicrobial action.

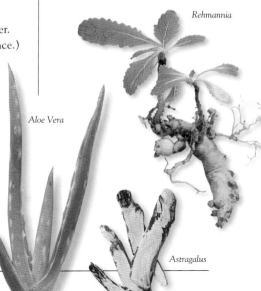

Rehmannia

Aloe Vera

Astragalus

How Aloe Vera works

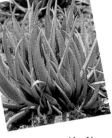

ABOVE *Aloe Vera can withstand harsh conditions.*

PRIZED BY THE *ancient Egyptians, Aloe Vera contains nearly 100 named constituents, of which 75 are active healing compounds. It can survive harsh conditions, including drought and radiation, and still do its healing work. It can treat a wide variety of internal and external problems, and can penetrate deeply into the skin and mucous membranes to soothe and fight infection.*

Two chemical aspects of Aloe Vera are used for medicinal purposes. Bitter Aloes are made from the dried, purified sap obtained from the latex – the thin layer of tissue directly beneath the skin. This bitter yellow substance contains resins, anthraquinones, and anthraglycosides, or aloins. It has a strongly purgative effect when taken internally and is usually used as a laxative. The latex is also used in after-sun products to soothe and moisturize.

It is the inner pulp of Aloe Vera that provides the juice and gel, which are most used for both internal and external healing. Anthraquinones, found primarily in the latex but also in small quantities in the gel, are to some degree responsible for Aloe Vera's anti-inflammatory and anesthetizing effects when applied to swellings, stings, sprains, and sunburn.

LEFT **The chemical components of Aloe Vera make it a highly effective healing plant.**

EXTERNAL USE

There are two theories to explain why Aloe Vera works externally. One is that it promotes rapid cell regeneration. The other is that Aloe Vera contains enzymes that cause chemical changes, thus intensifying healing.

The high water content of the gel (96%) carries nutrients to the site of external injuries. Although mainly water, the gel has the ability to lower the surface tension of water. When Aloe Vera gel or products are applied to the skin, the amino acids, vitamins, minerals, and other constituents are carried deep into the dermal layers to heal and soothe. Aloe Vera also eradicates dead skin cells, thus helping to regenerate cell growth and promote healthy tissue.

Although many claim that commercial products are more potent than the raw gel because they have higher concentrations of Aloe Vera's active ingredients, for most people the fresh gel gives excellent results. Aloe Vera gel appears to work best when applied from the leaf rather than removed and used alone.

RIGHT *Aloe Vera is applied to the skin externally in cream form.*

INTERNAL USE

Taken internally as a drink, Aloe Vera juice triggers a healing response for which a combination of constituents are responsible. The juice cleanses and detoxifies the digestive system, and thus influences other organs and systems. It contains magnesium lactate, which seems to lower stomach acidity, thus reversing the effects of indigestion and heartburn. It has proved to be very effective in the treatment of stomach ulcers; instead of reducing production of excess hydrochloric acid in the stomach as most ulcer drugs do, it coats the stomach lining.

BELOW *Aloe Vera is taken internally as a juice.*

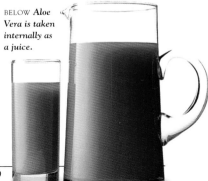

Aloe Vera can also raise hydrochloric acid levels. It is known as "amphoteric" (see page 56) because it can treat opposite conditions by raising or lowering levels of hydrochloric acid as needed (low hydrochloric acid levels are common and a contributing factor in allergies).

Aloe Vera restores balance in the digestive system in several ways. It acts as an alkalizing agent, it reduces yeast overgrowth, which destroys normal gut flora, and it penetrates the walls of the digestive system to remove harmful bacteria. Once balance is restored and beneficial flora reinstated, inflammation is reduced and the body is able to absorb nutrients. Painful disorders such as irritable bowel syndrome (IBS), acid indigestion, colitis, and Candida benefit from Aloe Vera.

By raising energy levels and promoting a sense of well-being, Aloe Vera reduces stress and tension, often the underlying cause of other complaints.

RIGHT **Aloe Vera promotes a sense of well-being.**

ALOE VERA'S EFFECT ON THE BODY

🌿 Cleanses and detoxifies, and is laxative but also remedies diarrhea.

🌿 Helps to boost and restore energy levels.

🌿 Supports the body's immune system.

🌿 Anesthetizes and cleanses damaged tissue and accelerates cell growth and regeneration.

🌿 Anti-inflammatory action helps to reduce heat and swelling, allowing natural healing to take place.

🌿 Restores levels of beneficial gut bacteria and stabilizes gastro-intestinal conditions.

🌿 Delivers complex nutrient compounds to all parts of the body, which in turn triggers specific healing responses.

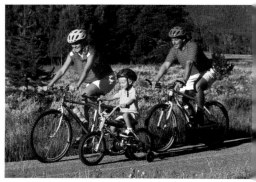

RESEARCH

Research into the natural healing properties of Aloe Vera has been carried out in Russia and the United States.

Medical and pharmaceutical research in Russia has been dictated by economic forces (plant medicines are less expensive than conventional drugs) and scientists there, to some extent, have been free of the pressures put on Western research scientists. For many years Russian scientists have been using Aloe Vera to treat patients suffering from diverse problems. For example, in addition to Aloe Vera's well-known benefits, Russian scientists have noted that it can bring about improvements in bone tuberculosis and broken bones; inflammatory gynecological conditions; paralysis caused by polio; ear, nose, and throat conditions, and bronchial asthma. They have also found that it can help retard the aging process.

Scientists in the United States and Russia have carried out extensive research into all types of burns including thermal burns. Aloe Vera contains an enzymatic property that, as well as healing the burn, is both cleansing and antibacterial. A cream has been developed in the United States containing 70% Aloe Vera juice extract, which prevents partially damaged tissue from dying and allows new epidermal skin cells to close off the area, thus promoting healthy new skin beneath the scab, rather than scar tissue.

Experimental research into the healing potential of Aloe Vera began in the United States in the 1930s in the search for a cure for radiation burns, but it developed into a pharmaceutical race to isolate the plant's active constituents, which could then be commercially reproduced to alleviate a wide range of conditions.

Finally, Aloe Vera has a role in the treatment of cancer. It seems that it causes the release of tumor necrosis factor Alpha, a substance that blocks the blood supply to cancerous growths. Also, a study at the University of Okinawa in Japan showed that drinking Aloe Vera juice regularly may be effective in preventing the onset of lung cancer in people who smoke.

International, scientifically validated research studies are continuing to make new discoveries into the effective applications of the healing powers of Aloe Vera.

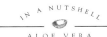
Conditions chart

THIS CHART is a guide to some of the conditions that Aloe Vera can treat, but it is not intended to replace other forms of treatment. Always consult your doctor or other qualified medical practitioner before embarking on a course of treatment. Follow dosages and application guidance given earlier in this book unless otherwise stated.

NAME	INTERNAL USE	EXTERNAL USE
ALLERGIES	Juice	
ABSCESSES AND BOILS		Gel, followed by cream
ACNE		Gel, cream
ARTHRITIS	Juice	Gel or cream
BEDSORES		Gel, powder
BRUISES		Gel
BURNS & SCALDS		Spray, gel followed by cream

NAME	INTERNAL USE	EXTERNAL USE
CANDIDA	Juice	Juice, gel or cream
CHICKENPOX	Juice	Gel, ointment
CHILBLAINS		Gel, cream
COLD SORES	Gargle	Gel
COLITIS	Juice	
CONSTIPATION	Juice	
CONVALESCENCE	Juice	
CYSTITIS	Juice	Gel or cream, douche
DANDRUFF		Gel
DIARRHEA	Juice	
EARACHE		Gel
ECZEMA	Juice, gel	Gel
EYES (IRRITATED)		Juice, diluted as an eyewash
GINGEVITIS	Gargle	

NAME	INTERNAL USE	EXTERNAL USE
HAYFEVER	Juice	
HEARTBURN	Juice	
INDIGESTION	Juice	
INSECT BITES AND STINGS		Gel
IRRITABLE BOWEL SYNDROME	Juice	
ITCHING	Juice	Gel, juice
MOUTH ABSCESS AND INFECTION		Gargle of mouthwash
PSORIASIS	Juice	Gel
PERIOD PAINS	Juice	
RHEUMATISM	Juice	Gel followed by cream
SHINGLES	Juice	Gel

NAME	INTERNAL USE	EXTERNAL USE
SKIN ERUPTIONS	Juice	Gel and ointment
SORE THROAT	Gargle juice before swallowing	
SPRAINS AND STRAINS		Gel, cream
STOMACH ULCERS	Juice	
SUNBURN	Poultice	Gel, cream
VARICOSE VEINS		Ointment
WOUNDS AND CUTS		Gel, cream

Glossary

ALLERGIC RHINITIS

An allergy to a number of everyday substances, such as house dust.

AMPHOTERIC

Ability of a substance to treat opposite conditions as required.

ANTIBACTERIAL

A substance that destroys bacteria.

ANTI-INFLAMMATORY

Reduces inflammation.

ANTIMICROBIAL

Destroys or inhibits the growth of microorganisms.

CAPILLARIES

The smallest blood vessels in the body, which carry blood in a fine network to all the body's tissues.

CHOLESTEROL

A fatty substance found in animal tissues and body fluids. A vital component of cell membranes, and especially of the myelin sheath that insulates nerves.

COLLAGEN

A protein that is the principal fibrous component of connective tissue in the body. It forms an important part of skin, tendons, and bones.

ENZYME

An organic catalyst composed mainly of protein found in all living systems, which is vital for the functioning of biochemical reactions.

FIBROBLASTS

A cell in connective tissue that is responsible for producing fibers.

FOLIC ACID

A member of the vitamin B complex occurring naturally in green plants, fresh fruit, liver and yeast. Now considered to be an important supplement during pregnancy.

HERPES ZOSTER

The medical name for shingles, an infection that results in a painful rash.

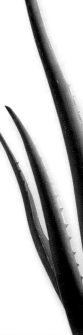

HOMEOSTASIS
Process of maintaining the body in equilibrium, despite external changes. Homeostasis is the primary aim of most organs in the body.

INTERLEUKIN
Defense enzyme produced by macrophages, cells that engulf toxins and tumor cells.

INTERFERON
A protein produced in response to an infectious virus, which stops the virus from replicating.

INULIN
Carbohydrate that stimulates the function of the immune system. It is filtered from the bloodstream by the kidneys, and tests for inulin are made to monitor kidney function.

IMMUNITY
Capacity and function of the body to fend off foreign bodies (fungi, bacteria, viruses), and/or to disarm and eject them.

LAXATIVE
A substance that stimulates the bowels to empty.

MACROPHAGES
Cells that are part of the immune system that destroy small particles, such as toxic chemicals and tumors. They are the deep cleansers of the immune system.

MUCOPOLYSACCHARIDES (MPS)
Any of the polysaccharides (group of sugars) that form chemical bonds with water to produce mucilaginous (lubricating) fluids. They also contain sugar derivatives such as amino acids.

PSORIASIS
A chronic skin disease in which scaly pink patches form on the scalp, knees, elbows, and other parts of the body.

TINCTURE
Remedy prepared by chopping up herb and soaking in a mixture of alcohol and water.

TOPICAL
A treatment that is applied directly to an affected area on the surface of the body as opposed to being taken internally.

VERRUCA
A fungal growth or wart on the sole of the foot.

Further reading

ALOE VERA HEALS, *Karen Gottlieb*, (Denver CO Royal Publications Inc., 1980)

ALOE VERA, JOJOBA AND YUCCA, *New Canaan, C. T.*, (Keats Publishing Inc., 1982)

A MODERN HERBAL, *Mrs. M. Grieve*, (Tiger Books, 1992)

AN ANCIENT EGYPTIAN HERBAL, *Lise Manniche*, (British Museum Publications, 1989)

BARTRAM'S ENCYCLOPEDIA OF HERBAL MEDICINE, *Thomas Bartram*, (Robinson, 1998)

BRITISH HERBAL PHARMACOPOEIA 1983 AND 1996 (British Herbal Medical Association, 1996)

THE COMPLETE BOOK OF HERBS, *Lesley Bremness*, (Dorling Kindersley, 1988)

THE COMPLETE ILLUSTRATED HOLISTIC HERBAL, *David Hoffmann*, (Element Books, UK, 1996)

ENCYCLOPEDIA OF HERBS AND HERBALISM, *Malcolm Stuart*, (Black Cat, 1987)

THE ENCYCLOPEDIA OF MEDICINAL PLANTS, *Andrew Chevallier*, (Dorling Kindersley, 1996)

THE ESSENTIAL BOOK OF HERBAL MEDICINE, (*Simon Y. Mills*, Arkana, 1993)

GARDENER'S DICTIONARY OF PLANT NAMES, *Dr. William T. Stearn*, (Cassell, 1983)

HERBAL GIFTS, *Jane Newdick*, (CLB, 1999)

HERBALGRAM, the journal of the American Botanical Council and the Herb Research Foundation

HERBAL HEALING FOR WOMEN, *Rosemary Gladstar*, (Bantam Books, 1994)

THE HERB SOCIETY'S HOME HERBAL, *Penelope Ody*, (Dorling Kindersley, 1995)

THE HOLISTIC HERBAL, *David Hoffmann*, (Element Books, 1988)

NATIONAL ALOE SCIENCE COUNCIL: *Brochures and quarterly publications*

NATURE'S PHARMACY: A HISTORY OF PLANTS AND HEALING (*based on the Pharmaceutical Society's Museum Collection at Kew Gardens*), *Christine Stockwell*, (Century/Hutchinson, 1988)

THE NEW GREEN PHARMACY, *Barbara Griggs*, (Vermilion Publications)

POTTER'S NEW CYCLOPAEDIA OF BOTANICAL DRUGS AND PREPARATIONS, (*R. C. Wren*, Health Science Press, 1973)

ROMAN GARDENS AND THEIR PLANTS, *Claire Ryley*, (Fishbourne Roman Palace, Fishbourne, undated, c. 1996)

SPIRITUAL PROPERTIES OF HERBS, *Gurudas*, (Cassandra Press, 1988)

TEXTBOOK OF MODERN HERBOLOGY, *Terry Willard*, (Wild Rose College of Natural Healing, Alberta, 1993)

Useful addresses

**British Herbal Medicine
Association (B.H.M.A.)**
Sun House, Church Street, Stroud,
Glos. GL5 1JL, UK
Tel: 011 44 1453–751389
Fax: 011 44 1453–751402
Association that works with the
Medicine Control Agency to
promote high standards of quality
and safety of herbal medicine

Herb Society
Deddington Hill Farm,
Warmington, Banbury,
Oxon. OX17 1XB, UK
Tel: 011 44 1295–692000
Fax: 011 44 1295–692004
Charity that disseminates
information about herbs and also
organizes workshops

SUPPLIERS IN THE UK

Baldwin & Company
171–173 Walworth Road,
London SE17 1RW, UK
Tel: 011 44 171–703 5550
Herbs, storage bottles, jars, and
containers available

East West Herbs
3 Neal's Yard,
Covent Garden,
London WC2H 9DP, UK
Tel: 011 44 171–379 1312
Suppliers of herbs and Reishi
mushroom powder

Hambleden Herbs
Court Farm, Milverton,
Somerset TA4 1NF, UK
Tel: 011 44 1823–401205
Organic herbs by mail order

Herbs, Hands, Healing
The Cabins, Station Warehouse,
Station Road, Pulham Market,
Norfolk IP21 4XF, UK
Tel/fax: 011 44 1379–608201
Organic herbal formulas;
Superfood; mail order and free
brochure also available

SUPPLIERS/SCHOOLS IN THE USA

American Botanical Pharmacy
PO Box 3027, Santa Monica,
CA 90408, USA
Tel/fax: 1310 453–1987
Manufacturer and distributor of
herbal products; also runs
training courses

Blessed Herbs
109 Barre Plains Road,
Oakham,
MA 01068, USA
Tel: 1800–489–4372
Dried bulk herbs are available by
mail order so that you can make
your own preparations

United Plant Savers
PO Box 420,
E. Barre, VT 05649, USA
Aims to preserve wild Native
American medicinal plants

*Other Healing Herb Books
in the Nutshell Series*

CRANBERRY
VACCINIUM MACROCARPON

HAWTHORN
CRATAEGUS MONOGYNA

ECHINACEA
*ECHINACEA ANGUSTIFOLIA
ECHINACEA PURPUREA*

MARIGOLD
CALENDULA OFFICINALIS

GARLIC
ALLIUM SATIVUM

MILK THISTLE
SILYBUM MARIANUM

GINGER
ZINGIBER OFFICINALE

ST. JOHN'S WORT
HYPERICUM PERFORATUM

GINKGO
GINKGO BILOBA

SAW PALMETTO
SERENOA SERRULATA

GINSENG
ELEUTHEROCOCCUS SENTICOSUS